OUTDOOR MEDICINE

MANAGEMENT OF WILDERNESS MEDICAL EMERGENCIES

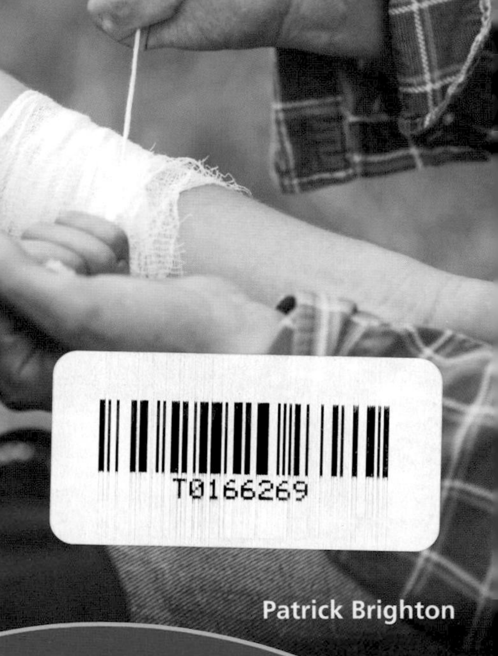

T0166269

Patrick Brighton

Adventure Skills Guides

CARE FOR CUTS, BRUISES, AND MORE

Adventure Skills Guides

The wild places on this planet represent one of the greatest gifts in life. Unfortunately, escaping to the wilderness also distances us from the advanced medical care available in urban areas. Rather than avoiding the backcountry for fear of possible medical emergencies, you can carefully plan your travels and arm yourself both with knowledge and the appropriate equipment needed to deal with any medical issues or emergencies that arise.

This guide is a template to help you provide appropriate field treatment for some of the most commonly encountered backcountry medical concerns and emergencies. Certainly no text can cover every possible emergency medical scenario; instead, this book is designed to help you logically think through an emergency and address your individual emergency situation.

PATRICK BRIGHTON, M.D.

Patrick Brighton is a board-certified general and trauma surgeon. A Fellow in the American College of Surgeons for 23 years, he has evaluated and surgically managed thousands of critically injured trauma patients, including those from dozens of mass-casualty situations. An avid alpinist and ice climber, Dr. Brighton currently spends most of his free time as a member of the Ouray Mountain Rescue Team in Ouray, Colorado. Dr. Brighton also teaches wilderness medicine courses in the U.S. and in South America.

Cover and book design by Lora Westberg
Edited by Brett Ortler

Cover image: **PRESSLAB/shutterstock.com**

All images copyrighted.

Used under license from Shutterstock.com
Africa Studio: 25; **Aleksei Ruzhin:** 6 middle; **Angel DiBilio:** 21; **Anukool Manoton:** 10; **astarot:** 3; **aSuruwataRi:** 13; **bubutu:** 7 middle; **CC7:** 30; **Chalamkhav:** 14; **Cristian Suciu:** 23; **Diederik Hoppenbrouwers:** 24; **Dudarev Mikhail:** 21; **Egor_Kulinich:** 5; **frantic00:** 10; **Ilya Andriyanov:** 11; **Jay Ondreicka:** 20 top; **Julian Popov:** 20 bottom; **Lithiumphoto:** 7 bottom; **Little stock:** outside flap; **Lorenzo Sala:** 12; **Lorraine Kourafas:** 22; **Mali lucky:** 8; **Microgen:** 5; **Mouy_Photo:** 18; **MriMan:** 14; **NaNahara Sung:** 15; **narin phapnam:** 17; **Nodty:** 4; **oumjeab:** 16; **Pan Xunbin:** 7 top; **pisaphotography:** 27; **pixelaway:** 26, 26; **robert cicchetti:** 29; **ShutterstockProfessional:** 6 bottom; **Steven R Smith:** 19; **systemedic:** 28; **THPStock:** 22; **Tim Mainiero:** 6 top; **Valik:** 9; **Vivienstock:** 19; **yhelfman:** 20 middle; **Zapylaiev Kostiantyn:** 18

10 9 8 7 6 5 4

Outdoor Medicine: Management of Wilderness Medical Emergencies
Copyright © 2019 by Patrick Brighton, M.D.
Published by Adventure Publications, an imprint of AdventureKEEN
310 Garfield Street South, Cambridge, Minnesota 55008
(800) 678-7006
www.adventurepublications.net
All rights reserved
Printed in China
ISBN 978-1-59193-851-4 (pbk.)

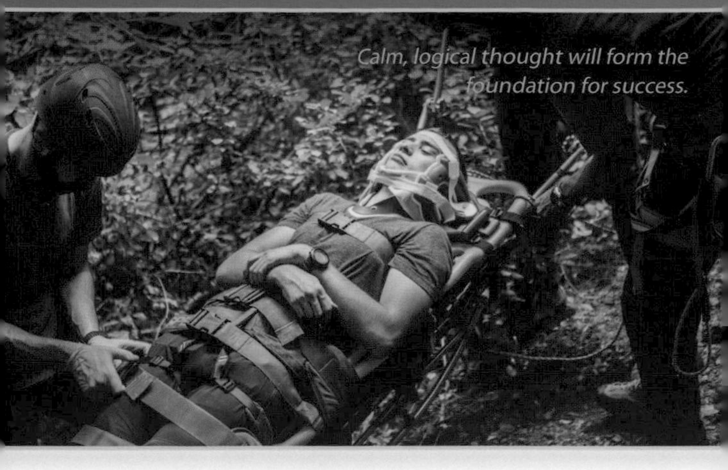
Calm, logical thought will form the foundation for success.

In the best of circumstances, managing a medical or trauma emergency can be one of the most stressful experiences a person can face. In a wilderness setting with limited resources and uncertain rescue possibilities, things become even more daunting, especially if one has just witnessed a family member or a friend suffer a critical injury.

The main goal of this guide is to provide you with the knowledge you'll need in an emergency; this, in turn, will help mitigate some of the stress you'll inevitably face in a real-life situation. Ideally, this guide is designed to be read completely before traveling into the backcountry, but its small size makes it easy to carry along as a quick reference.

In a catastrophic situation, it's crucial to make calm, logical decisions. That's why I teach three basic tenets when instructing students on how to cope during stressful medical emergency situations:

1) **You didn't do it.** Even on the off-chance that you did cause the situation, the only way to help is to forget that fact and focus on the solution. There will be plenty of time for retrospection later.
2) **No one dies in 2 seconds.** If someone dies within a very brief time, there is almost certainly nothing you could have done about it, so when confronted with a medical emergency, it is much better to take a moment and think logically about the best sequence going forward.

And probably most importantly:

3) **Do no harm.** Never make a decision that worsens the situation or the patient's condition, even if you are trying to save them in a heroic fashion. (This is the same principle behind the oath that all medical doctors take.)

1 HOW TO DO CPR

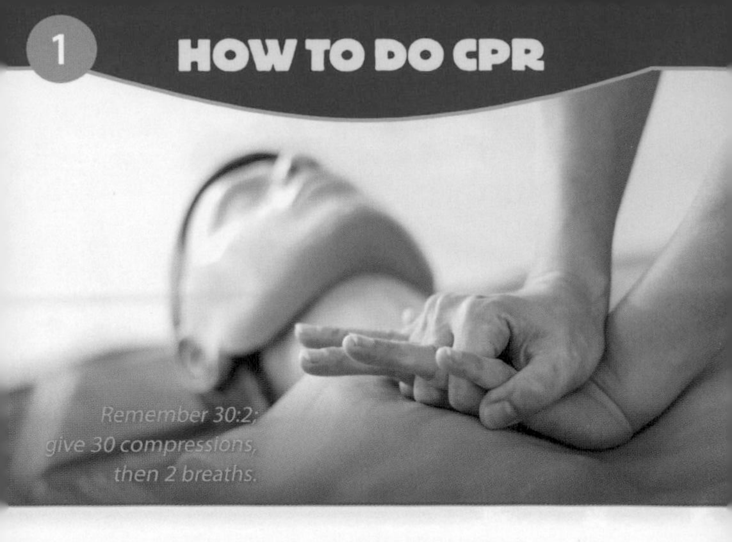

If an injury or illness is severe enough, it can cause a person's heart to stop and/or they may stop breathing. The treatment basics, regardless of cause, remain the same. Some of the most frequent backcountry causes of cardiopulmonary arrest are (1) heart attack (myocardial infarction), (2) lightning strike, (3) choking, or (4) trauma.

Cardiopulmonary Resuscitation (CPR)

As you evaluate a potential cardiopulmonary emergency, remember the ABCs: **Airway, Breathing, Circulation.**

Airway: If the person is unconscious, open their mouth and sweep to clear any foreign material. Make sure you don't push anything farther down the airway.

Breathing: Expose the chest. Examine it for chest rise/fall.

Circulation: Feel for a pulse. Taking an inguinal (groin) pulse is the most reliable pulse point.

Once you have established that the person has stopped breathing, that there's no obvious airway obstruction, and that they have no pulse, begin CPR immediately.

Chest Compressions/Rescue Breathing for an Adult

Place the patient on the hardest, flattest surface possible. If necessary, move the patient onto a flat surface, ensuring that spinal alignment is maintained. Have a partner hold the head still to prevent spinal cord damage in the event of a neck fracture. Then, pinch the nose closed and breathe forcefully into the mouth. Ensure you have a seal with the lips. Watch for the chest to rise. Give two breaths, then begin chest compressions.

To administer compressions, stack your hands, lock your arms, and bend at the waist. Place your hands at the center of the chest and press down. Compressions must be proportional to the patient's size. Adults will generally require about 2 inches of compression depth to provide adequate perfusion of vital organs. Compressions should produce a palpable inguinal (groin) pulse. Compressions should be 100 beats a minute for adults and children. A second rescuer may feel the inguinal pulse while compressions are given to gauge the adequacy of compressions. Having someone count the time with a stopwatch on a smartphone helps. After every 30 compressions, give 2 breaths. If two or more rescuers are present, try not to give a breath as the other person delivers a compression. Note that when performing CPR you are very likely to break the victim's breastbone and/or ribs.

Performing CPR on Toddlers/Infants

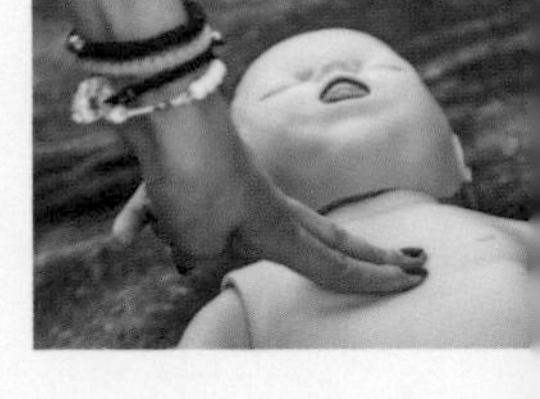

CPR on toddlers/infants follows the protocol for adults with the following differences: When performing rescue breathing, place your mouth over the victim's mouth and nose, and you also may be able to administer compressions with only one hand or several fingers. The goal is to compress just hard enough to circulate blood around the body, not damage the heart.

AEDs

Automatic External Defibrillators (AEDs) are portable devices used to detect abnormal cardiac rhythms and deliver shocks to restart the heart's electrical activity. One should be obtained as quickly as possible. Typically ranger stations, fire stations, etc., will have them available. Most search-and-rescue teams have them. CPR must be stopped briefly to place the AED. AEDs can be confusing to use, as each brand works slightly differently. Instructions are located on all brands. Basically, you place the two pads as directed (one over the heart, the other over the ribs on the patient's left side), and follow the prompts. Usually you have to hit the power button and then either follow the prompts or just hit the activate (or similar word) button. Sometimes no shock is delivered because the machine doesn't detect the appropriate cardiac rhythm to initiate the activation process. If the AED doesn't deliver a shock or if cardiac rhythm isn't re-established after three shocks, the chance for recovery is poor.

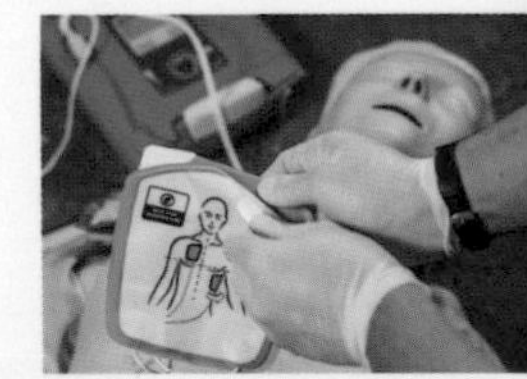

Take time to treat
small issues before
they become big ones.

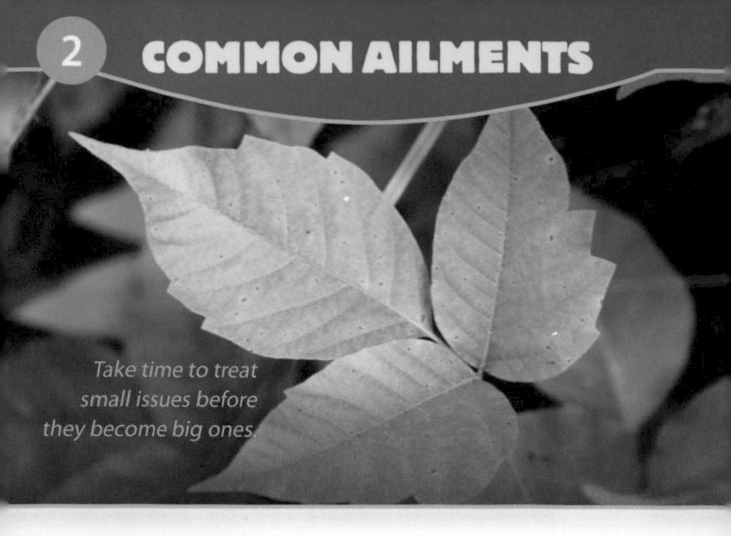

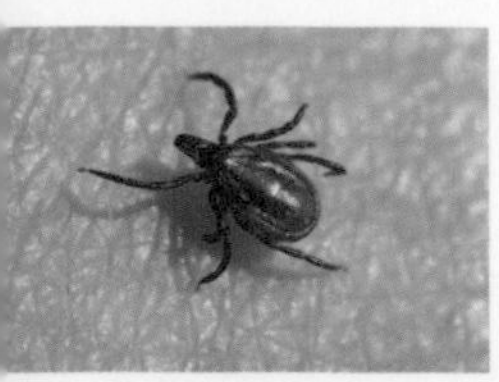

Insect Bites/Ticks

Non-venomous or minimally venomous bites from mosquitoes, chiggers, flies, etc., can be treated by cleaning with soap and water. Calamine lotion can be used for excessive itching.

Ticks can be removed by gently placing some sanitizing gel or rubbing alcohol on the tick and then grasping it as close to the skin as possible with a pair of sharp tweezers. Don't use blunt tweezers or you will just crush the body. Use gentle and constant pressure to remove it in its entirety. If the head breaks off, you can try to extract it with the tweezers. If you can't, it will usually heal fine anyway.

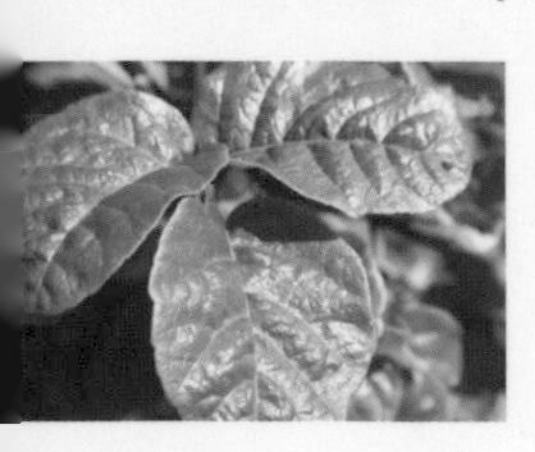

Contact Dermatitis

Plants such as poison ivy, poison sumac, and poison oak all produce a noxious oil called urushiol that triggers an allergic reaction in many people. Affected areas begin itching/ burning after 12–48 hours. Severe reactions can include extremely painful, raised, weeping blisters.

If you suspect you've come into contact with the plant, get away from it, and then change your clothes and wash any affected areas with soap. If this is done soon enough, the oil can be washed off. The oils are very adherent and hydrophobic (meaning water alone will not wash them off). Be sure to wash the clothing as well, with soap, as the oils can persist for great lengths of time. If a reaction is present, wash the affected skin with cool water, and wrap with a nonocclusive (breathable), non-constricting gauze wrap. Calamine lotion or a paste of cooked oatmeal (if in a remote setting) can provide some relief. These rashes usually take 1–3 weeks to resolve.

Slight Abrasions and/or Road Rash

Gently wash the wound with cool water. Only remove foreign material that is relatively easy to wipe away. Attempts to dig into the tissues can provoke a deep soft-tissue infection. For superficial abrasions, a scant amount of antibiotic ointment may help. Don't use any ointments for deep abrasions, as this may actually increase infection risk by trapping bacteria in a moist environment. Wrap loosely with dry gauze.

Blisters

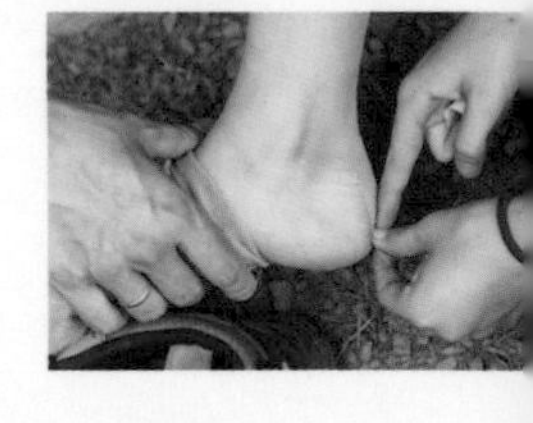

Blisters result from a continuous shearing force on the skin, such as a wet sock, a hiking pole, and so on. Prevention is obviously important; wear properly fitted footwear and gloves. When a blister forms, you may pop it to remove the fluid for comfort, but do not remove the overlying skin; it is protective and facilitates healing of the underlying raw tissue. Try to tape down the blistered skin to the underlying tissue with a Band-Aid and some tape, but don't make it too tight. If you have a foot blister, remedy the underlying problem by changing socks, adding socks, removing socks completely, or padding the interior of the shoe.

Larger Wounds/Lacerations

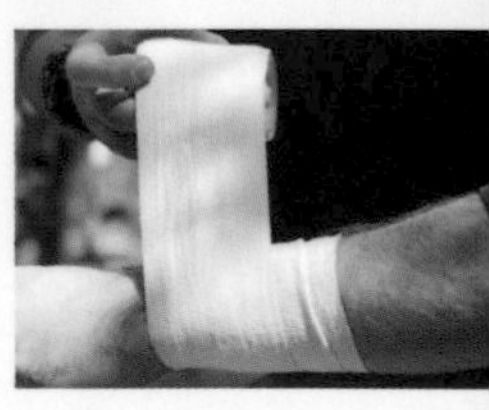

A laceration indicates a very thin, deep wound caused by a knife or similar object. The severity can range from a nuisance, such as a paper cut, to a life-threatening event, such as the transection of a major artery.

Stop the bleeding by applying direct pressure on the wound using the cleanest cloth available. This may require a prolonged effort. Severe arterial bleeding may rarely require a tourniquet (page 28). Once the bleeding is stopped, place a piece of gauze or the cleanest material available on top of the wound, and wrap it fairly snugly with gauze, an Ace wrap, tape, or whatever is at hand. It is vital to not wrap the wound so tightly that it impedes blood flow beyond the wound. If it is an extremity injury, check for a pulse at the wrist or the ankle. If an injury occurs that results in the loss of skin, underlying fat, or even muscle and fascia, and if closing it is impossible (even with sutures), get the patient to a hospital immediately.

Unless you are qualified to suture (sew up the wound) and have appropriate materials, lacerations should be treated like other wounds: Flush them with clean water, and use direct pressure to stop the bleeding. Many lacerations can be closed with tape. It is frequently possible to bring the tissues together with one hand (or a second pair of hands) and place a piece of tape perpendicular to the wound to keep it together. The patient should proceed to the nearest care facility; lacerations cannot usually be closed after 24 hours due to a risk of infection.

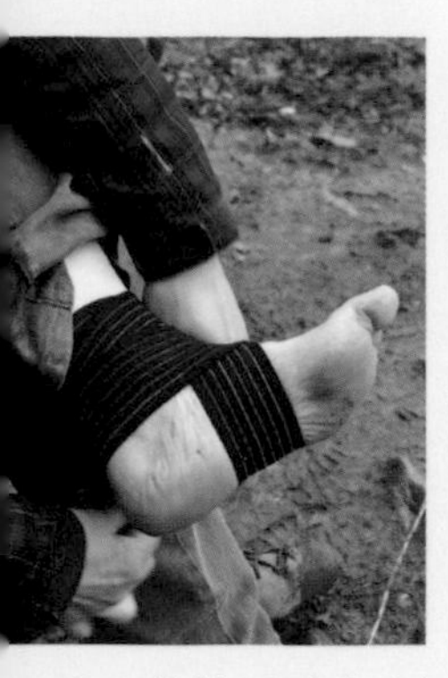

Sprains

Sprains are one of the most common soft tissue injuries in the backcountry. Technically speaking, a sprain is a sudden stretching (with associated microtearing) of the ligaments and tendons around a joint. Ankles are the most sprained joint. "Rolling an ankle" over a rock or another object is the usual culprit. After such an episode it is important to take care of the injury immediately.

Stop, remove the shoe, and elevate the foot above the heart. If a stream or ice/snow source is available, cool the joint. If it is imperative to continue walking, wrap the joint snugly, but not tight enough to impede blood flow, and lean on a companion or a walking stick. The treatments are similar for other joints.

Ibuprofen can help with the swelling and discomfort. In general, remember the mnemonic "RICE"– Rest, Ice, Compression (not too much), and Elevation. Sprains can be associated with fractures, so make sure to see a medical professional once you're back in civilization.

Stomach Problems and Gastrointestinal Infections

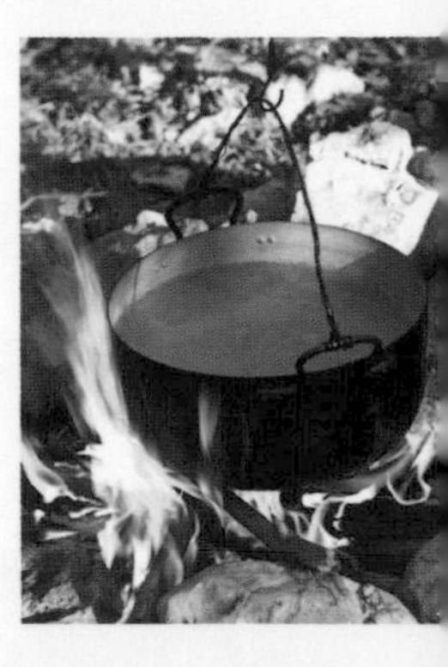

Nearly all gastrointestinal infections result from fecal-oral transmission—fecal material that is somehow ingested (often by drinking contaminated water). It is safe to assume that all water around the world is contaminated by one or more organisms that cause disease in humans, even if the water looks perfectly clear. Prevention, therefore, consists of purifying all water before drinking or cooking. Boiling water usually sterilizes things, but many organisms can survive in water up to 140–160 degrees Fahrenheit, and at high altitudes, water may boil at these temperatures. Filters or sanitizing tablets/drops work well if the directions are followed appropriately. Washing hands with soap and water and using an alcohol sanitizer are essential to preventing the spread of gastrointestinal infections. (Some organisms are killed by soap and water but not by alcohol and vice versa.)

All patients may lose a considerable amount of fluid through diarrhea and/or vomiting. Patients at either end of the age spectrum are especially vulnerable to the effects of dehydration, and if vomiting makes it impossible for a patient to drink, the situation may become life-threatening. Infants may die within only a few hours of ongoing, untreated fluid loss. In the elderly, such losses may produce electrolyte imbalances, which may lead to a fatal cardiac arrhythmia.

It becomes critical, therefore, to replace gastrointestinal fluid losses aggressively with copious water and electrolyte solutions. There are many powdered electrolyte solutions on the market; it is wise to carry some in the backcountry. A basic rule of thumb is to estimate losses through diarrhea and vomiting and replace it on a 2:1 schedule (i.e., 2 liters of oral intake for every liter of lost bodily fluid). Vomiting especially may deplete the body's reserve of potassium quickly, mandating rapid replacement of this electrolyte.

If a patient is unable to take oral liquids, evacuation must become even more of a priority.

EYE INJURIES

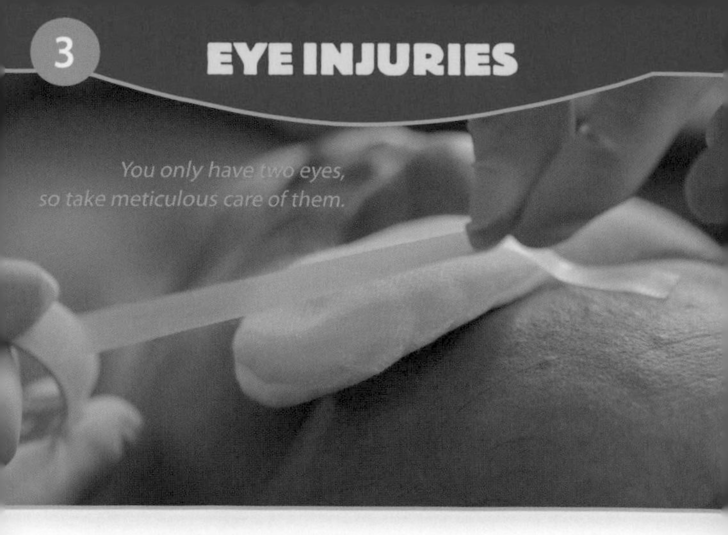

Corneal Abrasion/Laceration

The cornea is the exposed outer surface of the eye. Branches or wind-blown debris often cause corneal damage. Don't allow the patient to rub the eye; this worsens the injury. Position the patient on their back with the affected eye slightly closer to the ground. Wash the eye with clean water and with the eyelids held open. If antibiotic eye drops are available, place two drops in the affected eye, and cover it with gauze. If the patient doesn't need to see to travel, cover both eyes until they get medical help.

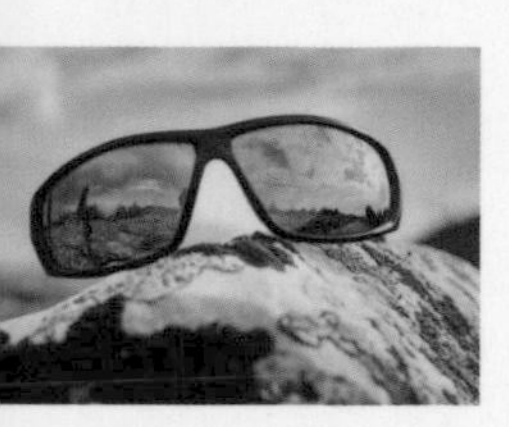

Retinal Burn

The retina is the back layer of the eyeball. Burns to the retina are usually caused by ultraviolet energy reflected off snow or water. Symptoms include severe eye pain, watering, headache, and temporary blindness. Remove the patient from the offending environment; place cool, moist cloths over their eyes; and let them rest. Keep the eyes closed until the pain subsides and vision returns. This might take several days. To prevent retinal burns, wear Category 4 wraparound sunglasses with both UVA and UVB protection. Goggles or glacier glasses should be used on snow.

Direct Trauma to the Eye

Penetrating or blunt trauma to the globe (eyeball) can be catastrophic and represents an extreme emergency. If there is a penetrating object, don't attempt removal. This can worsen the injury and may result in severe bleeding. Instead, cover both eyes, tape the object in place (the cut-off bottom of a plastic cup works), and arrange for rapid evacuation. For a complete rupture of the globe, surgery must be performed quickly to prevent the loss of the other eye due to a severe immune response.

NOSEBLEEDS

4

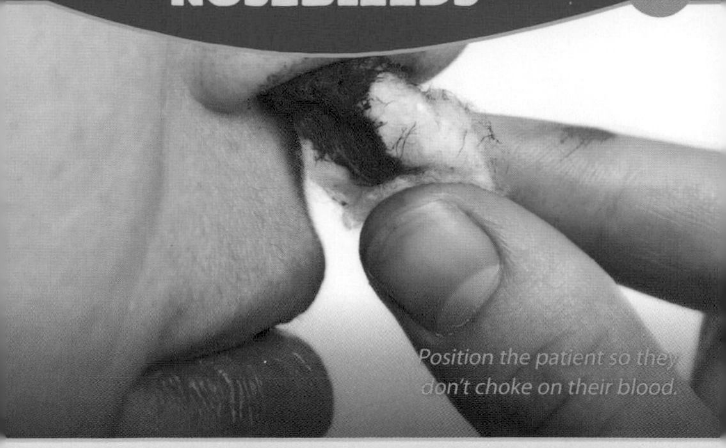

Position the patient so they don't choke on their blood.

Nosebleeds fall into two separate categories: anterior nosebleeds, which occur toward the tip of the nose and account for roughly 90 percent of nosebleeds, and posterior nosebleeds, which account for 10 percent of nosebleeds. While rare, posterior nosebleeds can be severe and even life-threatening. They result from the rupture of an artery in the back of the nose. They will usually not stop without significant intervention. Posterior nosebleeds can sometimes be distinguished from anterior ones by the increased volume of blood and occasionally by the brighter blood color. Usually, blood will pour down the throat, possibly causing choking and breathing difficulties.

Anterior Nosebleeds

Anterior nosebleeds are almost always easily treatable by tilting the head back and forcefully pinching the nose together. It may require 15 minutes or more for the blood to stop. Anterior nosebleeds are frequently caused by the drying out of the nasal mucosa (the mucous membranes that line the interior of the nose). After the bleeding stops, apply Vaseline or ChapStick inside both nostrils to moisten the mucosa and help prevent future episodes.

Posterior Nosebleeds

If you suspect a posterior nosebleed, keep the head above the heart level, and orient the victim's nose toward the ground. If you have a nasal tampon in your medical kit, use it. Pinching the nose together will not stop a posterior nosebleed. Instead, you'll need to evacuate the victim quickly, even if the bleeding stops, as it frequently recurs.

5 DENTAL EMERGENCIES

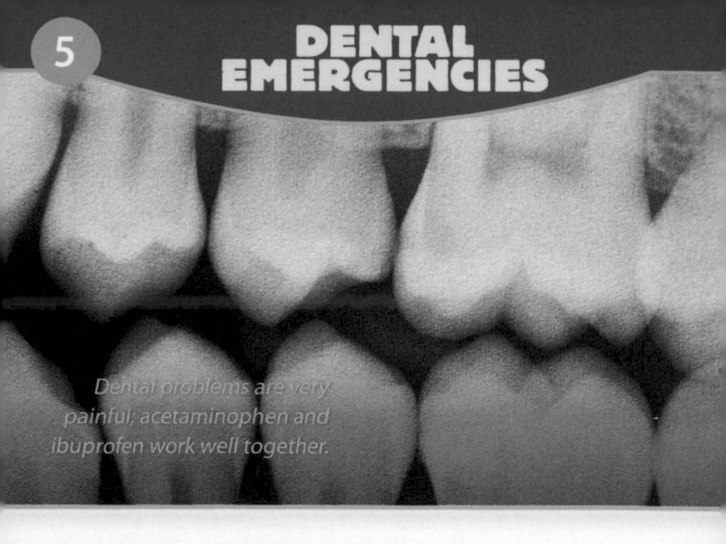

Dental problems are very painful; acetaminophen and ibuprofen work well together.

Dental emergencies typically consist of a lost filling or cracked teeth. Dental infections and abscesses can also occur, but they usually present over days to weeks and aren't often problems you will have to deal with in the backcountry.

Lost Filling

The loss of a filling will generally be felt as a sudden sensitivity to heat or cold. Even breathing ambient air can produce pain. Often this occurs during chewing hard or sticky food.

Saving the filling is usually unnecessary, as a dentist will remake it. If you carry a temporary dental filling paste in your medical kit, use it. After that, encourage the victim to eat soft foods, avoid chewing on that side, and visit a dentist as soon as possible. Clove oil can help with the pain.

Broken Tooth

When a tooth breaks, it is usually not a subtle phenomenon. Usually the patient hears a loud crunch while chewing a hard object. This is accompanied by excruciating pain as the sensory nerve of the tooth is exposed.

The treatment for a broken tooth is much the same as for a lost filling: Administer clove oil for the pain, eat soft foods, and avoid chewing on that side until the patient can see a dentist.

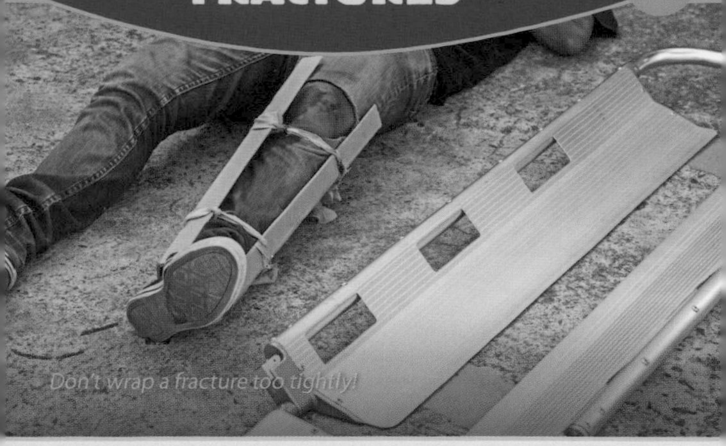

FRACTURES

6

Don't wrap a fracture too tightly!

Fractures

Fractures are divided into two broad categories: closed and open. The vast majority of fractures are closed fractures where there is no breach of the skin overlying the fracture. Open fractures represent a less common, but more serious, situation. Open fractures result when the skin is lacerated overlying the fracture site, regardless of whether the broken bone is visible. The laceration may be the result of a sharp, bony fragment piercing the skin or an external force that breaks the skin overlying the fracture. In either case, the result is the same: There is a serious risk of subsequent infection, the blood flow beyond the fracture may be compromised, and nerves located near affected arteries may be damaged.

The basic principles of fracture management are straightforward, but the specifics vary depending on the bone involved. Treatment essentially consists of immobilizing the fracture site, controlling any bleeding, and covering the open fracture with a clean, nonocclusive gauze. Pain control (ibuprofen works best) is also important.

Open fractures should be gently cleaned with clean water prior to bandaging and splinting the fracture. Water should not be forced into the wound, as this increases the risk of infection. Fractures should be splinted with rigid material wrapped by a non-constricting wrap.

If You Suspect a Fracture

1) Identify the fracture site–obvious by pain and swelling at the site.
2) Place rigid or semi-rigid objects on either side or loosely around the fracture site. Trekking poles, closed-cell sleeping pads, or tent stakes work well. Make sure to pad the area between the rigid object and the skin to prevent injury here.
3) Secure the rigid materials to the patient with gauze wrap, tape, cord, or similar material. Very important: Only wrap tight enough to keep the rigid material adjacent to the skin. Remember, the fracture site will continue to swell. The extremity must be periodically re-evaluated to ensure that the wrapping does not compromise the blood flow to the tissue beyond the fracture site.

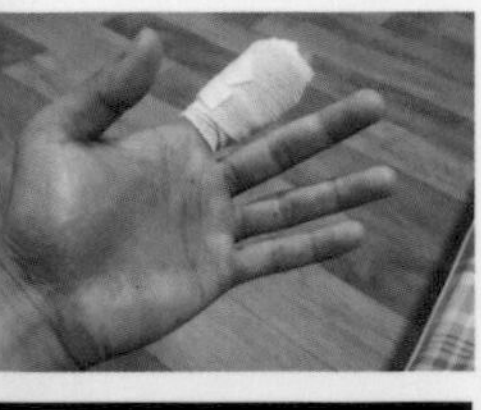

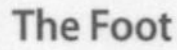

Fingers and Toes

These aren't usually terribly significant. Simply tape them loosely to the adjacent finger or toe.

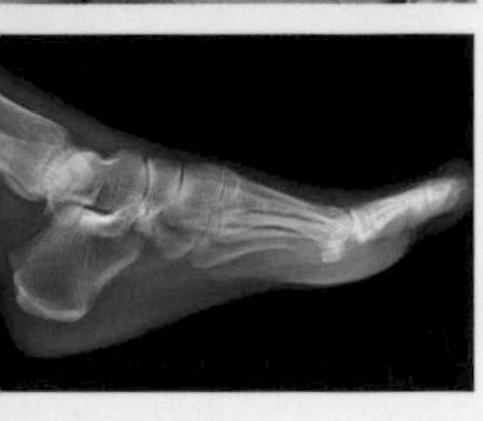

The Foot

There are many bones in the foot, and breaking one usually means the victim won't be able to walk. Immobilize the ankle joint in the position of maximum comfort. Make sure to check the toes periodically to ensure that the wrap is not too tight. The toes should have normal color and feeling.

Lower Leg

There are two bones in the lower leg: the tibia and the fibula. The fibula is on the outside of the leg; the tibia is more commonly known as the shinbone. The fibula provides minimal weight-bearing support; the tibia, by contrast, is one of the strongest bones in the body and supports essentially all body weight during a normal walking stride.

If you suspect a tibial fracture (or you're not sure which bone is broken), do not attempt to have the victim put weight on the leg. Instead, immobilize the ankle, knee, and fracture site, and evacuate them without having them bear weight on their leg.

For a fibula fracture, start by immobilizing the ankle, knee, and the fracture site. While not recommended, if you place a little weight on the fibula while evacuating the victim, it usually won't make things worse.

Femur

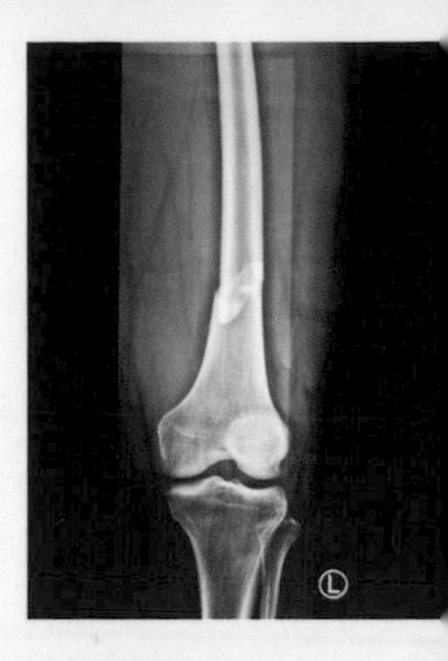

The long bone of the upper leg, the femur is a very strong bone surrounded by some of the largest muscles in the body. It takes a tremendous force to break; therefore, a broken femur represents a serious situation. It is possible to lose several units of blood (a unit is about a pint) into the soft tissues. A broken femur requires immobilization of the entire leg, along with the torso. Helicopter evacuation would be appropriate.

Compartment Syndrome

Major fractures of the extremities may produce such a large amount of swelling of the soft tissues that the limb's arteries are blocked and can no longer supply oxygen and nutrients to the extremity. This represents a true emergency; if not treated by a surgeon within a few hours, the limb—and possibly the patient's life—may be lost. This condition can be recognized by a tense, swollen extremity, mottled skin (blue and white discoloration), and the absence of a pulse in the hand or foot.

Pelvis

The pelvis is a ring of bone. Just as with femur fractures, pelvic (hip) fractures result from tremendous external forces. Crush injuries, falls, high-speed vehicle crashes, or similar forces are required. Because the pelvis is a rigid ring, it essentially always breaks in two or more places when a fracture occurs. Because of this, pelvic fractures can result in life-threatening blood loss.

Signs and symptoms of a broken pelvis include pain in the hip and/or lower abdomen, bruising and/or distension of the lower abdomen, and sometimes blood at the tip of the urethra. Arrange evacuation immediately by the quickest method available.

Field treatment consists of wrapping a sheet or towel around the pelvis as tightly as possible. Make sure that the wrapping material is not narrow, like a cord or webbing, to ensure that damage to the soft tissues does not occur. Raising the legs does not provide benefit and actually may worsen the blood loss.

Ribs

Simple rib fractures do not require treatment in the field besides pain medication and evacuation. Wrapping anything around the chest only impairs breathing and increases the risk of pulmonary infections. Oxygen may be helpful during transport.

If four or more contiguous ribs are broken in two or more places, what is known as a "flail chest" may occur. When this happens, the fractured segment bellows out paradoxically when the remaining chest bellows in and vice versa. This requires emergency evacuation, as respiratory failure may ensue quickly. A non-circumferential (i.e., don't wrap anything all the way around the chest) bandage taped in place may help limit the paradoxical movement and improve respiratory mechanics. To do this, cover the flail segment with gauze or whatever is available and then tape in place by taping along each of the four sides of the bandage. Remove the bandage if the respiratory status worsens.

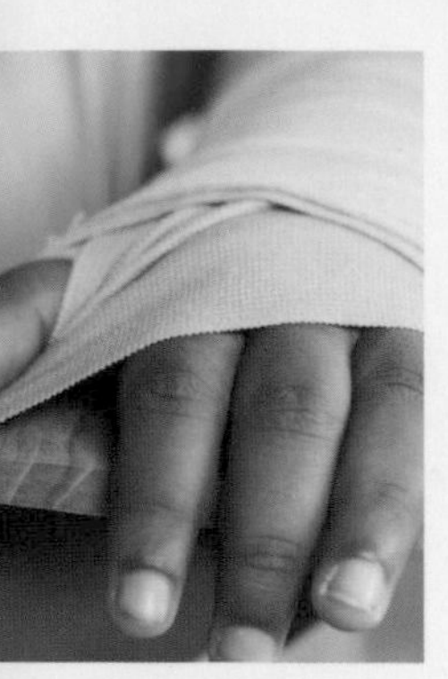

Hand/Arm/Forearm

Treat exactly like the corresponding bones in the leg (pages 14-15), i.e, the humerus is treated similarly to the femur, forearm similar to lower leg, hand similar to foot. Hand fractures must be immobilized to the forearm. Fracture of either forearm bone (radius or ulna) requires immobilization of the wrist and elbow as well. Upper arm (humerus) fracture necessitates immobilization of the entire arm, including the elbow. A triangular sling around the neck should be used after immobilization of the arm. Remember to check for pulses in the hand and evaluate for possible compartment syndrome (page 15).

Face/Skull

These always represent a serious injury. Do not attempt any field treatment aside from direct pressure to stop bleeding and arranging for a rapid evacuation.

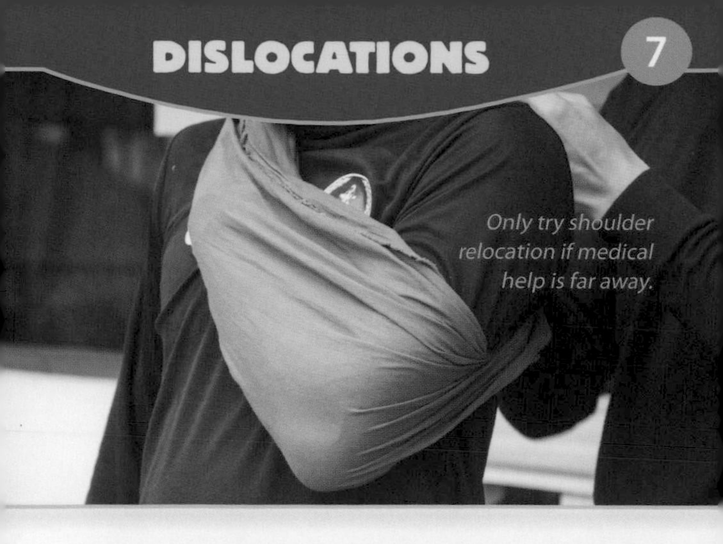
Only try shoulder relocation if medical help is far away.

Dislocations occur when a bone is forced out of its normal position in a joint. Ball-and-socket joints, such as shoulders, along with fingers and toes, are the most frequently dislocated joints.

All joint dislocations cause pain and swelling, and they are frequently associated with fractures of the bones within the joint, so it is not recommended to relocate a joint in the field. Definitive medical care, including an X-ray, must be performed as soon as possible. Remember, if you decide to relocate a joint in the field and you cause additional injury in doing so—you are responsible for that injury.

Shoulder

Far and away the most common dislocation, shoulder dislocations usually result from falling on an outstretched arm. In approximately 90 percent of shoulder dislocations, the humerus pops to the front of the body (an anterior dislocation). Dislocations with the humerus toward the back of the body indicate a posterior dislocation.

In general, it is best to have a professional relocate the joint with appropriate sedation and monitoring, but if definitive medical care is delayed, you may be forced to help a victim relocate it.

Multiple methods have been described to relocate anterior shoulder dislocations. Two of the most reliable methods are described here. The first method requires two rescuers. The first rescuer is positioned behind the victim with a sheet around the patient's torso (to hold the patient in place); the second firmly grasps the patient's wrist with one hand and the elbow joint with the other. The motion to relocate the joint is to pull the arm towards the rescuer who is doing the pulling, while at the same time gently externally rotating the arm (rotating the wrist away from the body). The most important aspect is to pull the arm away from the patient's body. Frequently, the joint will relocate without any rotation of the arm at all.

Alternatively, the patient may lie face-down on a table or on a very large rock, etc., with the injured arm dangling down. Tape empty water jugs or water bladders to the wrist and slowly fill them with water. This is a more consistently effective and gentle method than the first. Again, definitive medical care must be sought.

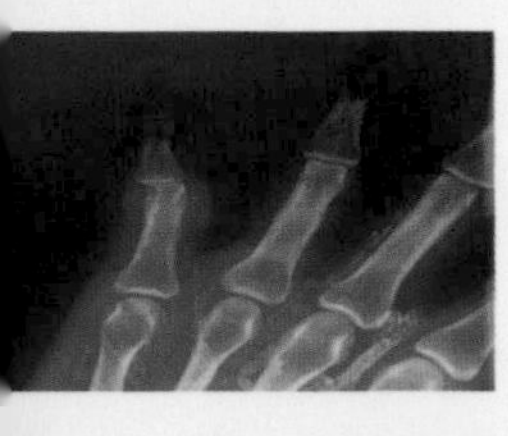

Fingers/Toes

It doesn't take much force to dislocate fingers or toes. If it is deemed necessary, it is usually possible to relocate the joint in the field by pulling on the end of the digit while guiding the bone back into place. If not successful, tape it to the adjacent finger or toe and seek medical care.

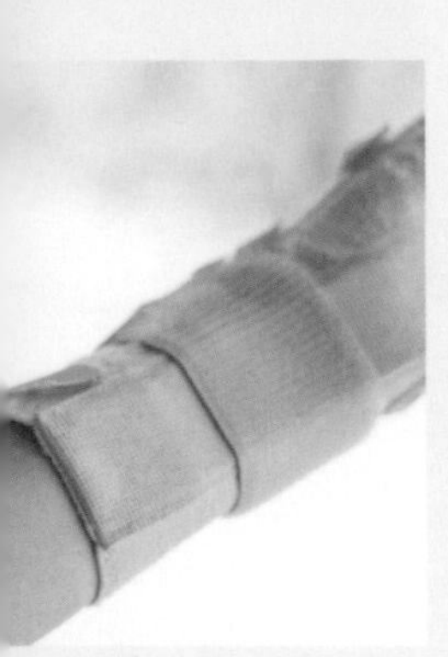

Ankle/Wrist

It requires a significant force to dislocate these joints, and dislocations are commonly associated with fractures. Splint in a position of maximum comfort and evacuate.

Knee/Elbow

It requires even more force to dislocate these well-supported joints, and dislocations are usually associated with fractures. Knee dislocations, in particular, often result in neurological and/or vascular injury.

For an elbow dislocation, the pulse in the hand should be monitored; for a knee dislocation, monitor the pulse in the foot. In either case, splint the joint in a position of maximum comfort and evacuate.

Hip

The hip joint is also a ball-and-socket joint, but due to the extremely large and powerful muscles that keep it in place, it requires extraordinary forces to dislocate, usually a significant fall or a motor vehicle accident. Dislocations are extremely painful and almost always accompanied by fractures of the pelvis.

The victim will exhibit a shortened, internally rotated (pigeon-toed) leg. Splint the extremity as for a femur fracture (include the hip and knee joints), and evacuate the patient ASAP (see pages 14-15 for details).

ANIMAL BITES

8

Take a photo of spiders and snakes that have bitten someone.

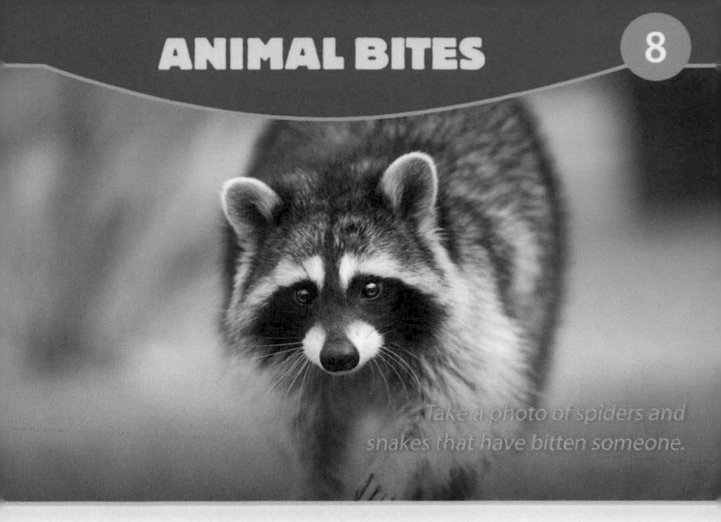

Animal bites and injuries represent unusual but potentially serious and even fatal events. Virtually all negative wild animal/human interactions result from inappropriate human behavior. Don't approach, feed, or otherwise position yourself too closely to any wild animal. Typically, animals view humans as prey only if the animals are old, infirm, injured, or have been fed by humans in the past.

Rabies

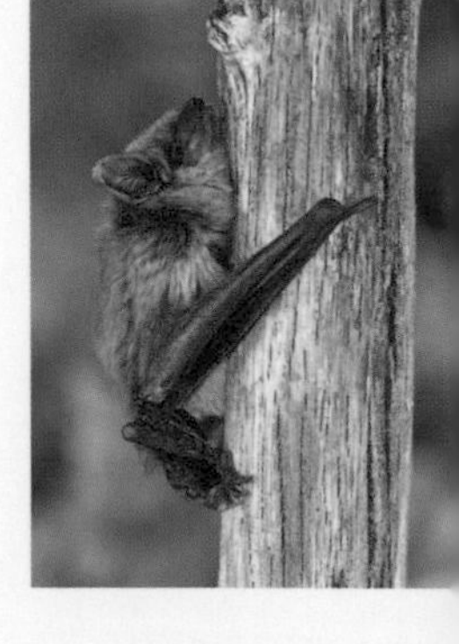

Rabies is arguably the most important concern for wild animal bites. Coyotes, foxes, skunks, bats, and raccoons are the most frequent carriers of the rabies virus. Any bite from a wild animal should be considered a rabies transmission event until proven otherwise. Left untreated, rabies is essentially 100 percent fatal.

If possible, kill the animal that bit the victim, but only attempt this if it's easy to overpower (such as a bat). It can then be tested for rabies. If the animal cannot be tested, the victim must receive rabies vaccinations immediately to prevent the full-blown expression of the disease. Field treatment of a bite or a scratch is to wash with clean water, direct pressure to stop bleeding, dress the wound with a clean dressing, and seek immediate medical care.

More serious bites, such as from a bear or a mountain lion, often result in significant blood loss and require immediate evacuation. Massive bleeding may require a tourniquet (page 28).

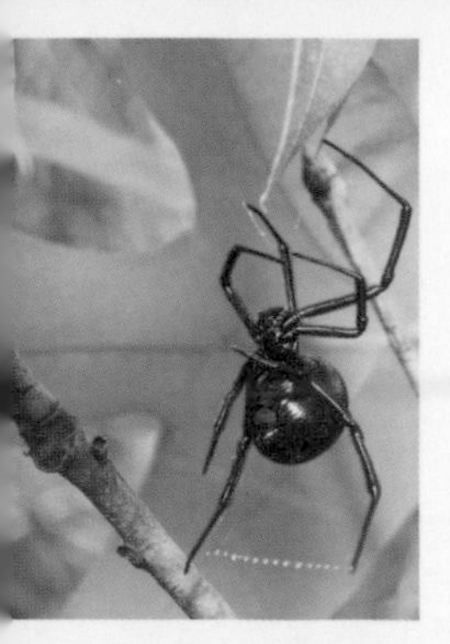

Bites and Stings from Dangerous Arachnids and Snakes

In the U.S., only two spiders—the black widow and the brown recluse—pose a threat to humans. Management includes a photo of the spider, elevation, ice, ibuprofen, and definitive medical care.

With few exceptions, venomous snakes in the U.S. belong to the pit viper family. Rattlesnakes, water moccasins (cottonmouth), and copperheads kill their prey by injecting venom through hollow fangs similar to hypodermic needles. Although rare, the amount of venom injected by a defensive bite may prove fatal to humans. Children are especially at risk due to their small size.

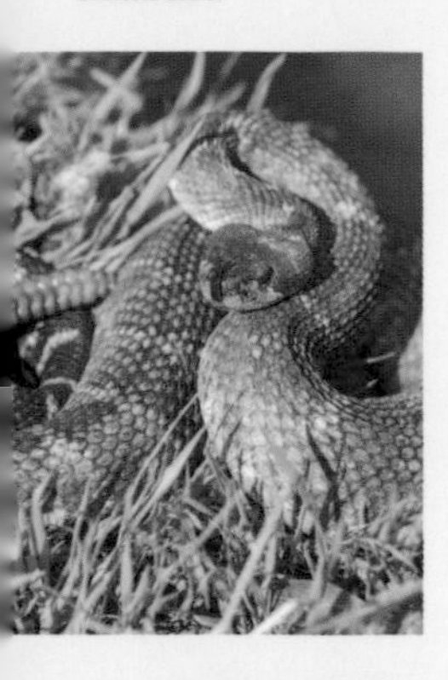

First, it is critical to identify the offending animal. A smartphone is the best way to do this. This evidence can be absolutely life-saving, as it can help doctors choose the correct antivenin to give in the emergency department.

For envenomations, some of the most critical points to consider are what not to do. Do not make a cut over the bite and try to suck out the poison. This does not work and may lead to serious injury and/or infection. Do not place a tourniquet; this provides absolutely no benefit, and the patient may well lose the extremity. Instead, limit the patient's activity, elevate the affected part, and transport the victim immediately to the nearest hospital.

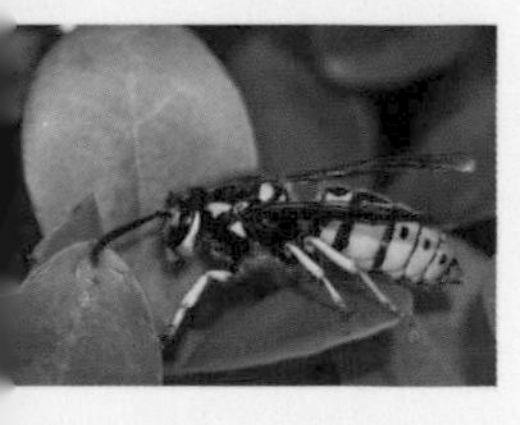

Anaphylactic Reactions

Severe, life-threatening allergic reactions are possible when bites or stings occur. They are typically the result of bee or wasp stings, but reactions to snakes, other animals, and even foods (such as peanuts) are possible too. If you suspect an anaphylactic reaction, administer an EpiPen and call 911. Instructions are printed on all EpiPen devices sold in the US, but basically expose the needle, jab sharply into the deltoid muscle or buttocks muscle, and push down the plunger until the syringe is empty.

DEHYDRATION & HYPERTHERMIA

9

Don't travel without adequate water!

Dehydration

We have all experienced dehydration on a hot day. The signs/symptoms of this mild form of dehydration include diminished salivation, thirst, and a rapid heart rate and breathing. Worsening of dehydration includes headache, diminished urine output, delirium, and, if left untreated, kidney failure, coma, and death. Obviously, prevention and early treatment are key.

Mild dehydration responds to oral fluids. It is important not to allow the person to drink an excessive amount of water (say, more than 3–4 liters) without an electrolyte drink of some sort. This can dilute the sodium content in the bloodstream and, in extreme cases, lead to seizures and death. To avoid this, alternate between water and an electrolyte drink. Severe cases will require intravenous fluids and transport to a hospital.

Hyperthermia

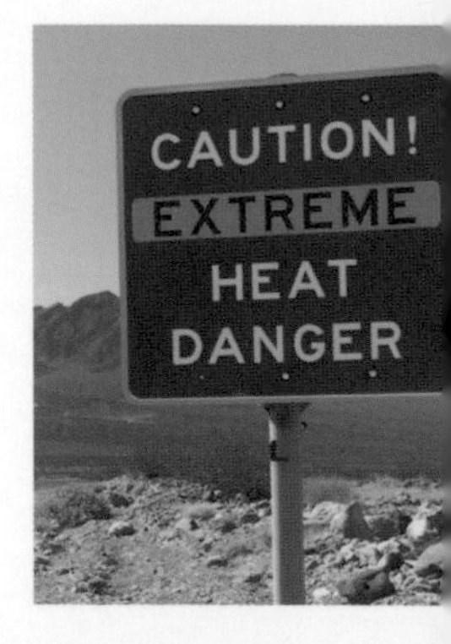

Once referred to as heat stroke or heat exhaustion, hyperthermia is a more descriptive term and indicates a patient with a rising core body temperature. The cause may be environmental (lost in the desert) or internal (fever). In a wilderness setting, environmental conditions are a much more common cause of hyperthermia than internal ones.

The normal human core temperature is 98.6 degrees Fahrenheit, plus/minus 0.2 degrees. In a hot environment, i.e., greater than 99 degrees, the body begins to attempt to dissipate

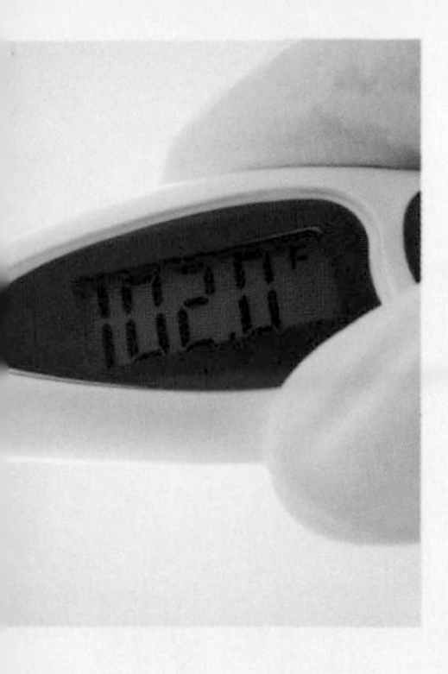

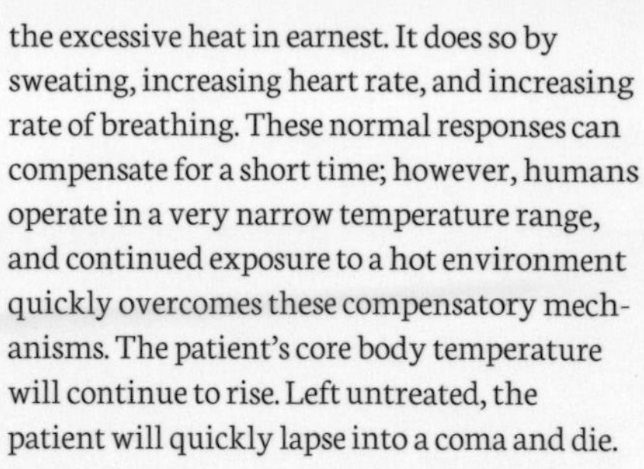

the excessive heat in earnest. It does so by sweating, increasing heart rate, and increasing rate of breathing. These normal responses can compensate for a short time; however, humans operate in a very narrow temperature range, and continued exposure to a hot environment quickly overcomes these compensatory mechanisms. The patient's core body temperature will continue to rise. Left untreated, the patient will quickly lapse into a coma and die.

Once a person's core body temperature reaches 106 degrees due to environmental causes, it is very difficult to salvage them, even in a hospital setting.

Treatment includes removing them from the hot environment and cooling them with water. Taking a cool bath or wiping exposed skin continuously with a wet rag will help. If they can drink, cold fluids will help. Regardless of the severity, patients must receive professional care immediately, as a relapse of symptoms often occurs, along with the insidious onset of organ damage.

FROSTBITE & HYPOTHERMIA

10

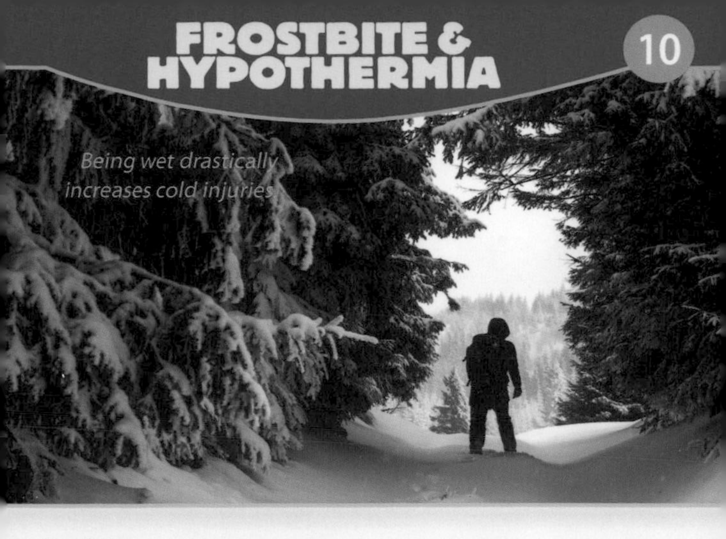

Frostbite

Frostbite occurs when tissues freeze. Frostbite does not usually occur with ambient temperatures above 10 degrees Fahrenheit, unless the skin becomes wet. Frostbite may occur in this setting at higher temperatures. Tissues farthest from the heart are at greatest risk for freezing (fingers, toes), as well as exposed areas (nose, cheeks). In cold environments, all skin must be covered, and frequent assessment of the at-risk tissues mentioned above must be performed. This includes removing boots/socks periodically to assess the circulation of the feet. Frostbite can be gradual and difficult to detect, and permanent tissue damage can occur before the patient is aware of it. When tissues freeze, a bluish discoloration marks the beginning of the process, followed by blistering. Much later (days to weeks), permanently destroyed tissue will turn black and die.

When frostbite occurs, treatment involves immediately stopping the freezing process and then rewarming the frozen tissues. Rewarming is best done with moist heat. A continuous warm bath of water between 100-103 degrees Fahrenheit works best. It is critical to not burn the fragile tissues, as even greater losses may occur. It is surprising how much tissue may be salvaged by expeditious treatment. Thoroughly dry the rewarmed areas and wrap with clean gauze to complete the field treatment. The patient must be transported to a hospital as quickly as possible. Frostbite occurs much more frequently at high altitudes, and the patient must be transferred to lower elevations as soon as possible. Oxygen delivered by mask may help oxygenate and preserve borderline viable tissue.

Hypothermia

Hypothermia occurs when a patient's core body temperature drops. The human body operates in an extremely narrow temperature range, and a decrease of even 1 or 2 degrees can be serious. When the outside temperature exceeds the ability of a person's clothing to contain their body heat, the core temperature begins to drop. Moisture accelerates this decrease dramatically. Hypothermia can be described as mild, moderate, or severe.

Mild: Core body temperature 93–97 degrees Fahrenheit. Symptoms include shivering, cutaneous vasoconstriction (contraction of the skin's blood vessels to conserve heat), and increased heart rate and breathing.

Moderate: Body temperature 88–93 degrees Fahrenheit. Increase in the mild symptoms, along with confusion, slurred speech, and clumsiness.

Severe: Body temperature below 88 degrees Fahrenheit. Symptoms can shift to slowed, shallow breathing; decreased heart rate; severe confusion; and drowsiness. The end stage of hypothermia can produce a paradoxical cutaneous vasodilation (expansion of the skin blood vessels), coma, and death. This can occur at any point below about 88 degrees Fahrenheit, but below 75 degrees Fahrenheit, death is common.

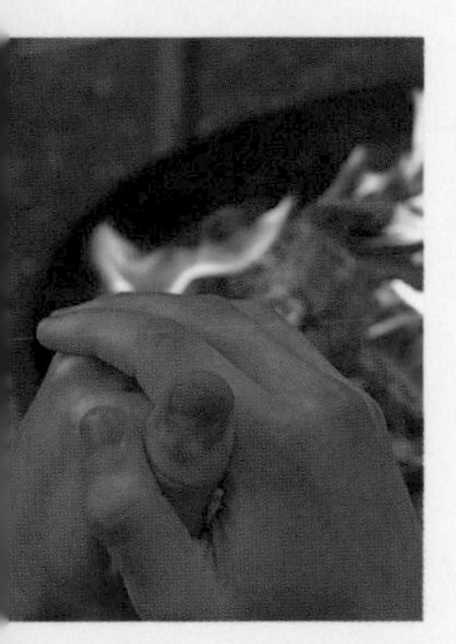

Treatment consists of removing the patient from the cold environment and removing all wet clothing. Even slightly damp clothes can make rewarming efforts very difficult. Hot water bottles (don't burn the skin!) placed in the groin area and armpits, skin-to-skin rewarming, and hot drinks (if conscious) all work well. Make sure to insulate the patient from the ground if unable to evacuate to a warm environment.

BURNS

11

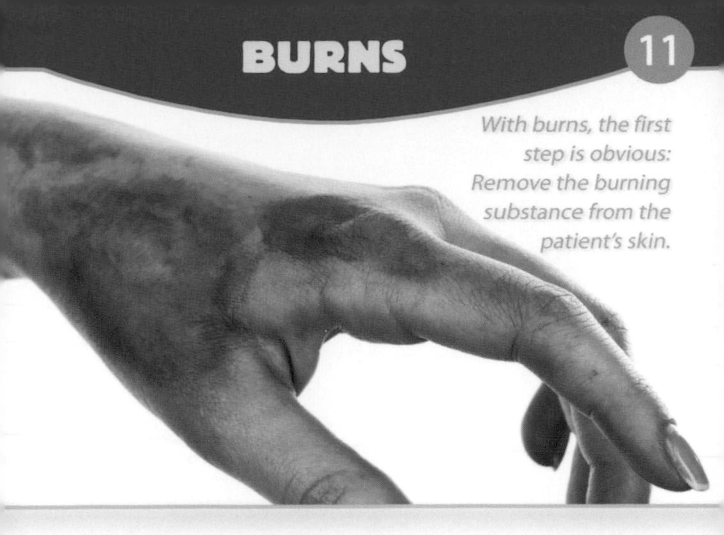

With burns, the first step is obvious: Remove the burning substance from the patient's skin.

Burns are not particularly common in the wilderness setting; in general, there are four types of burns.

First-degree burns: These affect only the outer layer of the skin (the epidermis). Another word for this condition is sunburn.

Second-degree burns (superficial partial thickness): These burns affect the outer layer of skin (epidermis) and into the inner layer (dermis).

Third-degree burns (deep partial thickness): These affect all layers of the skin and continue into subcutaneous fat.

Fourth-degree burns: These result from lightning strikes or electrocutions; the thermal damage includes all deep tissues, including muscle, fascia, even bone.

With the exception of first-degree burns, all burns lead to swelling, the loss of body fluids through the wound (blisters or weeping), and a systemic inflammatory response. When severe, loss of fluids can be massive, even life-threatening. All burns, other than first-degree, of any significant size must be managed in a specialized burn center. To estimate the size of the burn, use the patient's palm as a sort of tape measure. The palm represents about 1 percent of the surface area of a person's skin. Estimating how much of the patient's skin is burned is helpful to transmit to rescue personnel.

Field treatment starts with eliminating the source of injury, then removing clothing in the affected area and washing the burn with clean, cool water. Chemical burns must be washed for at least 10 minutes. Do not place any sort of salve on the burn, as this may increase the risk of infection. Wrap the burn very loosely with clean gauze. The burn area will swell massively, so a wrap that's too tight may lead to circulation compromise of the tissues beyond (distal to) the burn.

MEDICAL EMERGENCIES

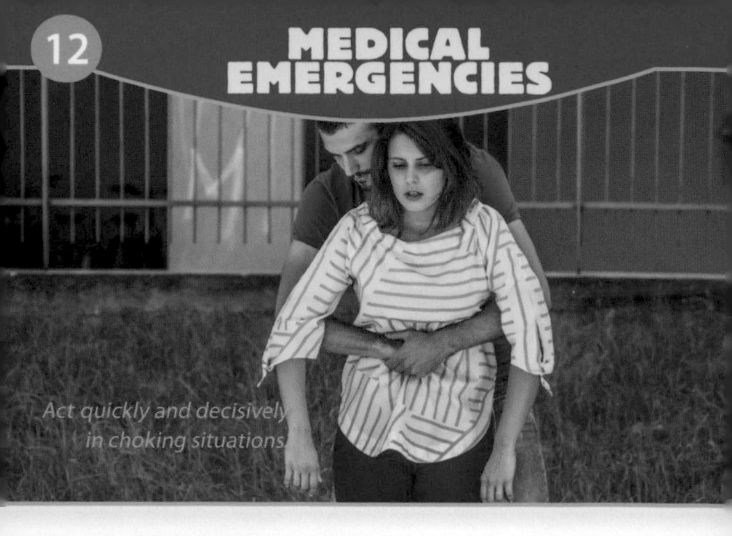

Act quickly and decisively in choking situations.

The Heimlich Maneuver

Choking occurs when foreign material is blocking the airway. Food is the usual culprit, but other material can become lodged in the back of the throat as well. For adults, the Heimlich Maneuver works best.

To perform the Heimlich Maneuver, stand behind the upright victim, place one fist directly below the sternum with the other hand stacked on top, and when the victim exhales, pull as sharply and forcefully as you can. It should almost feel like striking a blow. It must be as hard as you can, as there is a lot of tissue between your hands and the patient's diaphragm (the target). This may even break ribs or the sternum, but that can be dealt with later. Repeat until the material is dislodged. **Children** who are choking may be managed in a similar fashion. Choking **toddlers or infants** are treated by turning them upside down with the help of one or more rescuers and striking a sharp blow between the shoulder blades until the object is expelled. Use only the minimal force required to clear the airway to avoid injury to the victim's back or spinal cord.

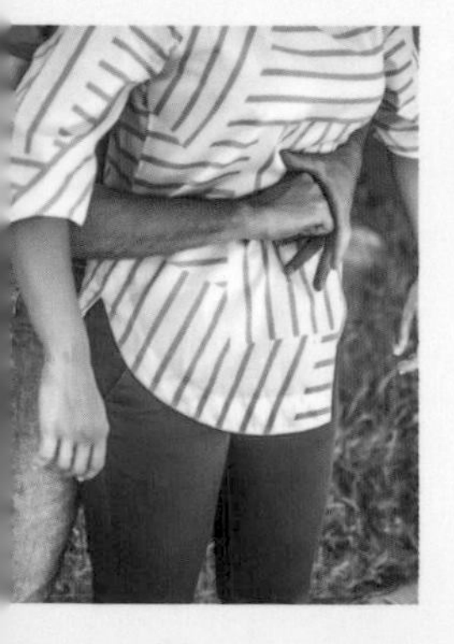

If a patient is too large to hold upright or wrap your arms around, another method exists to help expel a trapped foreign body in the airway. For the first, have the patient lie supine (facing skyward). Straddle the patient at the upper thighs, and stack your hands together with straight arms just as in preparation for CPR. Place the hands on the abdomen just below the breastbone. When the patient attempts to exhale or cough, thrust very forcefully at a 45-degree angle, aiming for a point on the floor between the upper shoulder blades.

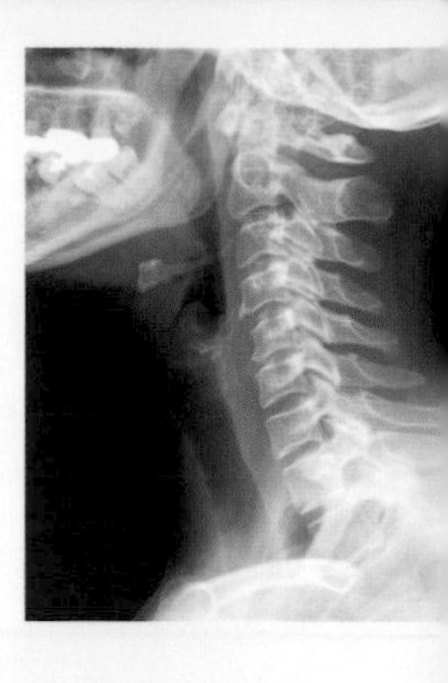

Spinal Cord Injuries

Spinal cord injuries represent a true emergency, and the patient must be transported to the nearest hospital as soon as possible. Signs and symptoms of spinal cord injury include pain at the injury site, "bogginess" (when the site is gently palpated it feels like kneading raw dough), and a loss of sensation or movement below the injury. Field treatment consists of addressing associated injuries and stabilizing the spine in a straight line. Any movement of the patient must be done by three or more rescuers. The patient can then be "log-rolled," with one person supporting the head and neck, with the rest rolling the body as a unit. Do not strap the patient firmly to a hard spine board. There is no need, and damage to the tissue over pressure points may occur.

Essentially all spinal cord injuries are associated with fractures and/or dislocations of the vertebrae at the injury site. These will produce extensive swelling at the site, as well as spasms of the surrounding muscles; this will act as an "auto-splint" of the injury. Because of these factors, conscious patients will not move their spines, so aggressive immobilization is unnecessary. Unconscious patients will require more care for immobilization but still do not need to be tightly compressed to a hard spine board.

A paradoxical situation occurs with spinal cord injuries above the lumbar level. For most trauma situations, a patient may become hypotensive (low blood pressure) with a rapid heart rate. With a spinal cord injury, patients frequently exhibit low blood pressure with a low heart rate. This is due to the severing of nerves that help to maintain blood pressure. In the absence of blood loss from additional trauma, this does not need to be treated aggressively. The information should be noted and transmitted to the appropriate medical personnel.

Spinal cord injuries at the cervical (neck) level may produce an imminently life-threatening situation. The nerves that control the breathing muscles originate from the spinal cord at this level, and transection of the cervical cord may result in respiratory failure and death within minutes. Unfortunately, without advanced life-saving equipment, not much can be done to salvage the victim.

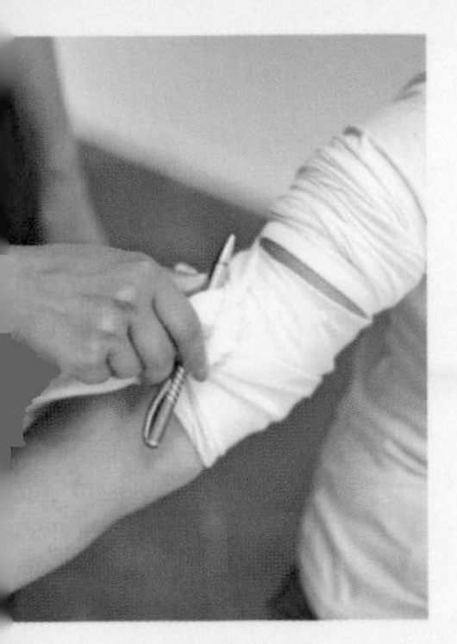

Massive Hemorrhage (Blood Loss)

Almost all bleeding can be stopped with direct pressure on the bleeding site. With a clean cloth and gloved hands, if available, press down firmly and directly over the bleeding site(s). Do not press anywhere but on the injury site. Maintain pressure on significant bleeding sites and arrange for the fastest possible transfer to a hospital.

To stop bleeding on an extremity, you can wrap one or two hands around the limb at the bleeding site and squeeze fiercely. Blood vessels become larger the closer they are to the torso; therefore, upper arm and leg bleeding requires considerably more force to stop. Unfortunately, not much can be done for internal bleeding of the chest or abdomen. Internal pelvic bleeding can be addressed with a very tight pelvic binder (page 15).

Tourniquets are a difficult topic. Placed correctly, they can be lifesaving. Placed incorrectly, they can be limb- or life-threatening. Tourniquets should only be placed in extreme circumstances where direct pressure on the wound fails to stop the bleeding. Place the tourniquet as close above the wound (between the wound and the heart) as possible. Tighten using the tension bar, but only until the bleeding stops! Write down the time the tourniquet was placed directly on the tourniquet (papers tend to get lost, and you might not accompany the patient to the hospital). Tourniquets left in place longer than two hours may make the limb unsalvageable. Tourniquets should only be loosened in a hospital setting by a trauma surgeon.

Before you try to use a tourniquet, make every attempt to stop bleeding with direct pressure. In the lower extremity below the knee, there are three main arteries. Bleeding from one of these can be impressive, but it can essentially always be stopped with moderate pressure. If a tourniquet is injudiciously placed, the other two normal arteries will be blocked along with the damaged one, and the extremity will completely lose blood supply. A similar situation occurs in the forearm.

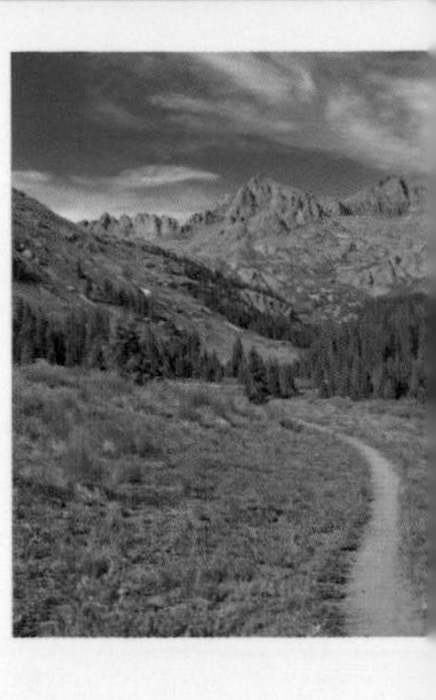

High-altitude Illnesses

Visitors to areas with high elevations (generally 10,000 feet above sea level or more) may suffer from a number of signs and symptoms collectively known as Acute Mountain Illness (AMS) or High-altitude Illness (HAI). Problems typically arise when people ascend faster than 1,000 feet (300 meters) per day or ignore early symptoms. The onset of HAI is unpredictable. Even seasoned mountaineers who have summited Mount Everest have developed HAI on subsequent forays, sometimes at much lower elevations.

High-altitude diseases usually start with a headache; it usually manifests as pounding pain in the temples but can also occur as a severe pain in the back of the skull. If untreated, the process may progress into High-altitude Cerebral Edema (HACE), High-altitude Pulmonary Edema (HAPE), or both.

HACE occurs when fluid accumulates within the brain. This swelling impairs normal brain functions, notably cognition and movement. Patients become confused, disoriented, and mumble incoherently. As the brain swells, it's pushed up against the hard skull, leading to walking difficulties (ataxia). The victim will stumble as if drunk and will eventually be unable to walk. Any or all of these latter symptoms indicate the end stages of the disease; death is imminent if left untreated.

HAPE represents the same process as above, except in the lungs. The lungs fill with fluid, and the patient begins to gasp for air and displays very rapid, shallow breaths. The accumulating fluid causes them to cough and leads to ruptured blood vessels in the lungs, which produces the classic end-stage symptom of the disease: a bloody, frothy sputum. Once a patient progresses to this stage, mortality is very high, even with treatment.

Prevention is key to avoiding both conditions. If someone is ascending at over 8,000 feet above sea level and a headache strikes, have them stop immediately and descend. On the way down, have them drink a liter of water or another liquid. If a patient develops any symptoms of HACE or HAPE, treatment must be immediate and decisive: They must descend immediately, under their own power or not. They should drink fluids if able. Oxygen should be administered by a high-flow mask. Dexamethasone should be administered by mouth or by injection (by qualified personnel only). As treatment and descent occur simultaneously, evacuation should be arranged.

Perhaps one of the most disconcerting and emotionally damaging situations that can occur is the witnessing of a severely injured person. For any trauma other than straightforward and isolated injuries, I encourage everyone to remember the "ABCs."

A—Airway. Ask the patient their name. If they respond in a normally pitched voice, the airway is open. If they are unconscious or are not able to speak normally, place the patient on their side (taking care to keep the spinal column, including the head and neck, in a straight line), and carefully open the mouth and sweep it clean with a gloved finger. Sometimes a foreign body or the tongue may impede normal airflow.

B—Breathing. Evaluating someone's breathing is different than checking their airway. Expose the chest enough to visualize that both sides of the chest move with respirations. If the patient is awake and able to cooperate, ask them to take deep breaths. Observe each side of the chest to see if they move equally. Ask the patient if they feel they are able to breathe normally. If a stethoscope is available, use it to listen to the lungs from the back. You don't have to know what you are listening to necessarily; instead, describe what you're hearing (e.g., "equal breath sounds" or "one side sounds hollow" or "rapid and shallow.") This is important information to relay to medical personnel.

C—Circulation. Quickly assess the patient for any signs of massive, potentially life-threatening bleeding. To do this, you need to take off or look under the clothing; bleeding from extremity injuries is usually obvious, but bleeding within the abdomen or chest cavity can be extremely difficult to ascertain. Pulses should be felt in all extremities. If a blood pressure measuring device is available, use it. Record blood pressures on a cell phone or piece of paper at intervals, usually every 10 minutes or so for severely injured patients. Use a tourniquet if needed (page 28).

Remember to follow these steps in order **before** proceeding to the next. one. This sequence is important because airway issues will kill a patient more quickly than breathing issues, and breathing issues will generally be fatal before bleeding issues.

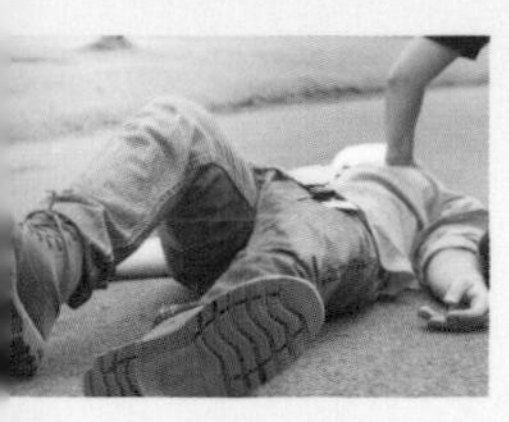

Only **after** the ABCs are evaluated and addressed should one proceed to a thorough, head-to-toe assessment of the patient. (Again, check underneath clothing.) The ABCs represent the only way to effectively manage a severely injured patient, and going through that simple and easy-to-remember mnemonic helps refocus the mind to the task at hand.